Nursing & Health Survival Guide

Dementia Care

Second Edition

Dawn Brooker, Sue Lillyman and Mary Bruce

T0298277

Second edition published 2023
by Routledge
4 Park Square, Milton Park, Abingdon, Oxon OX14 4RN

and by Routledge
605 Third Avenue, New York, NY 10158

Routledge is an imprint of the Taylor & Francis Group, an informa business

First edition published by Routledge 2013

British Library Cataloguing-in-Publication Data
A catalogue record for this book is available from the British Library

Library of Congress Cataloging-in-Publication Data
Names: Brooker, Dawn, 1959– author. | Lillyman, Sue, author.
Title: Dementia care / Dawn Brooker, Sue Lillyman, and Mary Bruce.
Description: Second edition. | Milton Park, Abingdon, Oxon; New York,
NY: Routledge, 2022. | Series: Nursing and health survival guides |
Includes bibliographical references and index. Identifiers: LCCN 2022004566 (print) |
LCCN 2022004567 (ebook) | ISBN 9781032217659 (spiral bound) | ISBN 9781003269946 (ebook)
Subjects: LCSH: Dementia–Nursing. | Dementia–Patients–Care. | Dementia–Treatment.
Classification: LCC RC521.B764 2022 (print) | LCC RC521 (ebook) |
DDC 616.8/310231–dc23/eng/20220217
LC record available at https://lccn.loc.gov/2022004566
LC ebook record available at https://lccn.loc.gov/2022004567

ISBN: 978-1-032-21765-9 (pbk)
ISBN: 978-1-003-26994-6 (ebk)

DOI: 10.4324/9781003269946

Typeset in Helvetica
by Newgen Publishing UK

Access the Support Material: https://apps.apple.com/gb/app/nursing-health-survival-guide/
id551297713

contents

Tables

Acknowledgements

Thanks to the Association for Dementia Studies team at the University of Worcester. Also, to our colleagues outside the university and to our family and friends who have enabled and continue to enable us to travel this journey.

1 Dementia Overview

■ NUMBERS, TYPES AND SYMPTOMS

- The number of people living with dementia in the UK is predicted to rise to 1.6 million by 2040 (Wittenburg et al. 2019).
- Worldwide the predictions are estimated at 131.5 million people by 2050 (Alzheimer's Society 2021).
- Dementia is an umbrella term for over 200 sub-types of progressive neurodegenerative disorders, which vary in their pattern of expression and neuropathy (Blossom and Brayne 2014). The most common ones are described in Table 1.1 below:
- Dementia symptoms include changes in thinking abilities (cognitive functioning), such as:
  - memory (disorientation and short-term recall)
  - communication (receptive and expressive dysphasias)
  - the ability to see the world as others do (visuo-spatial problems)
  - the ability to carry out practical everyday tasks (dyspraxias)
  - the ability to plan a course of action (dysexecutive syndrome)
  - problems with social control of behaviours (disinhibition).
- Diagnosis requires that more than one of these problems needs to be present and be sufficiently severe to impact on daily life.

DOI: 10.4324/9781003269946-1

Table 1.1 Percentage of dementias disease

UNDERLYING DISEASE	PERCENTAGE OF DEMENTIAS DISEASE ACCOUNTS FOR (%)
Alzheimer's-type dementia	50–75
Vascular dementia	Up to 20
Mixed (Vascular/Alzheimer's)	10
Dementia with Lewy Body	10–15
Fronto-temporal dementias	2
Parkinson's dementia	2
Other dementias	3

Alzheimer's Society (UK) 2021

- The dementias are progressive over time, beginning with subtle changes in behaviour but leading to severe disruption of function.
- The course of the progression depends on the type of dementia and on other physical, psychological and social factors for each individual.
- The label Mild Cognitive Impairment (MCI) is used when the individual experiences cognitive problems that are more advanced than those associated with normal ageing but are not severe enough to interfere with daily life.
- Individuals with MCI have an increased risk of progressing to dementia than other individuals of the same age without MCI.

- Dementia is not part of normal ageing, but the risk of getting it increases with age – see Table 1.2:
- Globally there is a new case every 3.2 seconds (Alzheimer's Disease International 2015).
- One in three people with Down's Syndrome develop Alzheimer's Disease in their 50s (Alzheimer's Association 2021).
- Other health factors associated with increased risk of dementia include stroke, Parkinson's Disease, head injury, diabetes mellitus and general cardiovascular risk factors (high blood pressure, smoking, high cholesterol, renal failure, family history).

(Alzheimer's Society (UK) 2021)

■ PERSON-CENTRED APPROACHES

- People living with dementia are at risk of their personhood being undermined and person-centred approaches to care were developed to protect against this (Kitwood 1997; Brooker and Latham 2015).

Table 1.2 Incidence of dementia in age ranges

AGE (YEARS)	INCIDENCE OF DEMENTIA
40–64	1 in 1,400
65–69	1 in 100
70–79	1 in 25
80+	1 in 6

Alzheimer's Society (UK) 2021

- SCIE Guidelines on Person Centred Care (2021) identified person-centred care as:
  - prompting service users as decision makers;
  - providing a service with the person living with dementia at the centre as an expert in their own experience;
  - recognising and taking into account the preferences and needs of physical comfort and safety;
  - emphasis on doing rather than doing to with the person playing an active part in the design and delivery of services.
    - People living with dementia should be viewed as individuals with autonomy, independence and the freedom to make their own choices.
    - They should have the opportunity to be actively involved in decision-making processes about polies and programmes, especially those concerning them.

For further information see the UN convention of persons with disabilities at: https://www.un.org/disabilities/docume nts/convention/convoptprot-e.pdf

■ NATIONAL DEMENTIA STRATEGIES

England, Wales, Scotland and Northern Ireland have all developed national strategies for the care of people with dementia, which are available as follows:

England: www.dh.gov.uk/en/Publicationsandstatistics/Publi cations/PublicationsPolicyAndGuidance/DH_094058

Wales: www.wales.nhs.uk/healthtopics/conditions/
dementia

Scotland: www.gov.scot/publications/promoting-excelle
nce-2021-framework-health-social-services-staff-work
ing-people-dementia-families-carers/

Northern Ireland: www.health-ni.gov.uk/sites/default/files/
publications/dhssps/improving-dementia-services-
2011.pdf

■ GUIDELINES AND WEBSITES

The Department of Health and Royal College of Nursing (2019) use the mnemonic SPACE to highlight the top five ingredients to support good dementia care:

Staff who are skilled and have time to care
Partnership working with carer
Assessment and early identification of dementia
Care plans that are person centred and individualised
Environments that are dementia friendly

Department of Health's (2010) 'Quality outcomes for people
with dementia: building on the work of the National
Dementia Strategy': www.dh.gov.uk/prod_consum_dh/
groups/dh_digitalassets/@dh/@en/@ps/documents/digit
alasset/dh_119828.pdf

Department of Health's 2011 'National Dementia Strategy,
Equalities Action Plan': www.gov.uk/government/publicati
ons/national-dementia-strategy-equalities-action-plan

Royal College of Nursing: www.rcn.org.uk/clinical-topics/
dementia/professional-resources

The 'Prime Minister's challenge on dementia', 2020: https://assets.publishing.service.gov.uk/government/uploads/system/uploads/attachment_data/file/414344/pm-dementia2020.pdf

National Institute for Heath and Clinical Excellence, Dementia Quality Standard 2019: www.nice.org.uk/guidance/qs184

NICE/SCIE joint publication: 'Dementia – Supporting people with dementia and their carers in health and social care': www.scie.org.uk/publications/misc/dementia

National Audit of Dementia Care in General Hospitals 2019: www.rcpsych.ac.uk/news-and-features/latest-news/detail/2019/07/10/national-audit-of-dementia-fourth-round-report-published?searchTerms=dementia%20care%20in%20general%20hospitals

Groups:
- Alzheimer's Disease International: www.alz.co.uk
- Alzheimer's Research UK: www.alzheimersresearchuk.org
- Alzheimer's Society: www.alzheimers.org.uk.
- Dementia Action Alliance: www.dementiaaction.org.uk
- Dementia UK: www.dementiauk.org

2 Communicating Well in Dementia Care

- People with dementia have particular challenges around communication. Taking time to communicate can make a real difference to how people feel and behave.
- The communication approach will depend on how impaired the individual's ability to communicate is.
- The aim is to find a response that supports the person with dementia while not undermining their remaining abilities.
- Some people – particularly early on in their dementia – may have very little problem communicating. It may be enough simply to be aware, and just to use conversational prompts such as regular summarising to help the person keep track.
- Others may have virtually no language at all and will need a lot more help to ensure their 'voice' gets heard. This group needs regular warm contact from staff but is often the group that receives least attention.

■ UNDERSTANDING COMMON COGNITIVE IMPAIRMENTS

- Cognitive disabilities are often misunderstood. Common misperceptions are that the person is being awkward, manipulative, attention-seeking, aggressive or ignorant. Appreciating that behaviours are caused by the person having unmet needs, and are not something within the active control of the person with dementia, is key to good communication.

DOI: 10.4324/9781003269946-2

- Dementia results in an increasing inability to express ideas through speech in a clear way.
- People lose the ability to communicate in languages that are not their mother tongue more quickly, even if they have been fluent in that language in adult life. The ability to understand language progressively worsens over time.
- Following instructions may be particularly difficult and can lead to frustration. Telling a person to move a particular part of their body may not be helpful. More helpful is to distract the person with conversation so that they can undertake the actions without thinking about them.
- Dementia often disables those parts of the brain that allow people to remember new events that have happened after the onset of the dementia. Even events that are very important, such as the death of a loved one, may not be remembered consciously or consistently. This is not to say that the event is not important to the person with dementia or that they do not have any memory at all of the event, merely that recalling it clearly can be difficult.
- Memories that have been there for many years, which developed before the onset of dementia, are usually clearer and seem much more present than recent ones.
- Misunderstandings can occur when the person is trying to make sense of what is happening by using long-held memories rather than recent events. For example, if a person with dementia finds themselves in hospital this may reawaken unpleasant memories of hospitalisations when they were younger.

- With visuo-perceptual cognitive problems, a person with dementia may literally see the world differently. Where others see a polished floor, the person with dementia may see a wet and slippery surface and where others see a sink, the person with dementia may see a toilet.

■ SPECIAL APPROACHES IN HOSPITALS

- Hospitals need to identify those patients with dementia to ensure their needs are met. Some have adopted a patient identification system, such as the 'Butterfly Scheme', and associated REACH guidelines to ensure good communication: www.dementiauk.org/what-we-do/uniting-carers/the-butterfly-scheme/
- Good communication is key to the Dementia Care Bundle approach, alongside nutrition, hydration and safe environment (Willoughby 2012).

■ THE VERA FRAMEWORK

Developed to guide everyday interactions of nursing staff (Blackhall et al. 2011), the mnemonic stands for:

Validation
Emotion
Reassure
Activity

The following case study demonstrates how this is used in practice:

Mary is sitting looking very tense and agitated in the chair next to her bed. When you ask her what is wrong, she tells you that she has to get home because it is getting dark now and her mum will be worried about her.

Possible responses:

- **Validation:** *'You sound ever so worried about that, Mary. Tell me about your mum.'* This addresses Mary's context, her rationale and perception of the problem is accepted and not questioned, and she is encouraged to say more about her perception.

- **Emotion:** *'I would feel worried too if I thought my mum didn't know where I was.'* This connects the healthcare professional to an empathic understanding of the worry that Mary experiences.

- **Reassure:** *'You are safe here, Mary. Everyone at home knows you are safe here.'* This simple statement of fact communicates the intention that no harm, real or imagined, will come to Mary.

- **Activity:** *'We are getting ready for having tea here now. Can you help me to put the water jugs on the trolley?'*

  An activity is constructed that fits with Mary's preoccupation that it is late in the day and that preparations need to be made for tea. It incorporates her behaviour rather than invalidates it.

■ NON-VERBAL COMMUNICATION

- There is no decline in depth of feeling or the range of emotions that people with dementia experience, even when verbal abilities have declined.
- As verbal abilities are lost the importance of warm, accepting human contact through non-verbal channels becomes even more important.
- If the professional's body language or facial expressions convey annoyance, this is what a person with dementia will notice, even if the words the professional is using are saying something very different.
- Attending carefully to the non-verbal behaviour of the person with dementia is important in assessing how the person is really feeling.
- Piecing together fragmented speech and summarising what has been heard is helpful to ensure understanding.
- When language has gone, there is a reliance on more fundamental non-verbal communication, such as touch, holding, stroking, eye contact, smiles and warmth.

3   Diagnosis of Dementia

- A large number of people still never receive a diagnosis of dementia, and the national dementia strategies seek to change this.
- Most people say they would like to know if they have a diagnosis of dementia because it puts them in a position to plan for the future. A small number say they would rather not know.
- A diagnosis of dementia needs to be based on a thorough assessment and it needs to be given in a sensitive and timely manner.
- Timely diagnosis is complex and it is recommended that this is undertaken by specialist mental health services based in memory clinics.
- Memory clinics usually take referrals directly from GPs and aim to give a rapid response and be non-stigmatising.

■ DIAGNOSTIC TESTS

- A full comprehensive physical and mental health assessment is recommended.
- A full history should rule out causes of delirium (acute confusion), such as infections, nutritional state, vitamin deficiency, thyroid problems, depression and side effects of medication; other mental health problems, such as depression; and other causes of neurological impairment.

DOI: 10.4324/9781003269946-3

■ MENTAL STATE EXAMINATION

Part of the assessment includes a mental state examination. Some of the more common tests are:

- Mini-Mental State Examination (MMSE), information available at: www.parinc.com/Products/Pkey/237
- General Practitioner Assessment of Cognition (GPCOG) Score, information available at: https://patient.info/doctor/general-practitioner-assessment-of-cognition-gpcog-score
- Abbreviated Mental Test (AMT), information available at: www.patient.co.uk/doctor/Abbreviated-Mental-Test-%28AMT%29.htm
- 7 Minute Screen™, information available at: www.verywellhealth.com/what-is-the-7-minute-screen-98636
- SLUMS Examination from St Louis University, information available at: www.slu.edu/medicine/internal-medicine/geriatric-medicine/aging-successfully/assessment-tools/mental-status-exam.php

■ INVESTIGATIONS

The following investigations should be carried out:

- routine haematology;
- biochemistry tests (including electrolytes, calcium, glucose, renal and liver function);
- thyroid function tests;
- serum vitamin B12 and folate levels;
- electroencephalography;

- MSU for delirium;
- temperature, pulse and respirations for infection;
- cerebrospinal fluid sample (only for people with CJD).

■ SUB-TYPES OF DEMENTIA

Once it is established that a dementia is present, it is now usual to diagnose the underlying disease process. There are over 200 types of dementia, most of which are very rare. The most common ones, together with their presenting symptoms, are described in Table 3.1 below. For fuller descriptions see Abou-Saleh et al. (2011) and Jacoby et al. (2008).

Table 3.1 Primary symptoms and types of dementia to consider

PRIMARY SYMPTOMS	TYPE OF DEMENTIA TO CONSIDER
Steady progressive loss of memory, language and functional disability Decline in the ability to reason Impaired visuo-spatial skills Poor judgement Attitude of indifference Reduced capacity to carry out activities of daily living	Alzheimer's Disease

Table 3.1 (*Continued*)

PRIMARY SYMPTOMS	TYPE OF DEMENTIA TO CONSIDER
Poor concentration and communication, and physical symptoms such as paralysis or weak limbs Physical signs of stroke	Vascular dementia
Insidious onset Recurrent visual hallucinations that involve vivid and colourful complex images of people or animals or other objects that may provoke emotional responses such as fear, amusement or indifference Insight into the unreality of the hallucination Auditory hallucinations, sleep disturbance Difficulty judging distances, impaired recent memory and fluctuating cognition with pronounced variation in attention and alertness Tremors	Dementia with Lewy Body

(*Continued*)

Table 3.1 (*Continued*)

PRIMARY SYMPTOMS	TYPE OF DEMENTIA TO CONSIDER
Changes in personality and behaviour, and emotional and language dysfunction but no dysfunction in memory Personality changes, progressive aphasia, impaired emotional and social functioning Behaviour manifestations including apathy, self-neglect, disinhibition, blunted effect, lack of insight, insensitivity to others Perseverative activity (clapping, humming, singing) Echoing words and phrases Excessive or compulsive eating or drinking Later stage: mutism, dysphagia, incontinence	Fronto-temporal dementia syndromes
Similar to AD but affects only memory with slower progression	LATE (limbic-predominant age-related TDP-43 encephalopathy)

Table 3.1 (*Continued*)

PRIMARY SYMPTOMS	TYPE OF DEMENTIA TO CONSIDER
Short-term memory loss and changes in mood such as frequent mood swings, depression, and feeling increasingly anxious, frustrated or agitated with increasing confusion and disorientation	Chronic Traumatic Encephalopathy
Rapid and progressive mental cognitive inability, visual loss, spasticity, myoclonic jerks and limb weakness Cortical blindness	Creutzfeldt–Jakob Disease
Impaired memory, planning, organising, judgement, social skills and balance	Alcohol-related brain damage

■ ALZHEIMER'S DISEASE (AD)

- Around 60 per cent of people diagnosed with dementia have Alzheimer's Disease. This is the most common type of dementia. Amyloid plaques and neurofibrillary tangles, mainly in the neocortex, block the transmission of signals from the neurons. AD symptoms correlate with reduced levels of acetylcholine.

- AD has been divided into different early presentations (McKhann et al. 2011):
  1 amnestic (primary impairment in memory plus another cognitive impairment);
  2 executive dysfunction (primary impairment in reasoning, judgement);
  3 Posterior Cortical Atrophy (PCA) (primary impairment in spatial cognition);
  4 language presentation (primary impairment in word finding).
- Rare in people under 65 years of age, early onset (40–50 years) is linked to genetic factors – for example, an inherited form called Familiar Alzheimer's Disease (FAD) caused by a faulty gene and also people with Down's Syndrome
- There is increased incidence in people who have a first-degree relative with AD, but this may be due to environmental rather than genetic factors.
- Three to seven stages are described, although these are not distinct and there are many individual differences.

Early stage

People in this stage may:

- be unable to recall recent conversations or events;
- repeat themself in conversations;
- be unable to follow conversations;
- be slow at grasping new ideas;
- demonstrate poor judgement;

- have difficulty in making decisions;
- lose interest in activities and/or people;
- blame others for their mistakes;
- be resistant to change;
- become agitated, distressed when unable to recall, remember or manage tasks.

Middle stage

People in this stage may:

- now forget conversations, places and appointments;
- be unable to recognise people;
- confuse generations;
- forget to take care of personal hygiene;
- forget to dress or go to the toilet;
- be disorientated in time and place;
- have difficulty with perception;
- confuse day and night;
- get easily upset;
- become easily upset or angry;
- lose confidence.

Late stage

People in this stage may:

- be unable to recognise people, objects and places;
- be frail, unsteady on their feet, prone to falls and eventually immobile;
- experience difficulty with eating and swallowing;
- eat excessively;

- lose or gain body weight;
- be incontinent;
- be restless, distressed and/or agitated;
- lose the ability to speak.

■ VASCULAR DEMENTIA (VaD)

VaD is the second most common type of dementia.
- It is also sometimes referred to as multi-infarct dementia.
- It is caused by ischaemia, anoxia or hypoxia of the brain resulting in brain damage and is associated with cardiovascular and cerebrovascular disease.
- Risk factors include:
  - smoking
  - raised blood pressure
  - serum lipids
  - high dietary fat intake
  - abnormal insulin metabolism
  - head trauma
  - environmental toxins.
  - Dementias associated with cerebrovascular disorders are potentially preventable and modifiable by preventing new infarcts.
  - VaD can present in different ways early on and diagnosis can be complex (Gorelick et al. 2011).

■ MIXED DEMENTIA (MD)

The most common is a combination of AD and VaD.

- Any combination of dementias can occur.
- A person with mixed dementia will experience a mixture of the symptoms of the dementias they have.
- Mixed dementia is much more common in those over 75 years.
- If a person has mixed dementia the progression appears more rapid.

■ LEWY BODY DEMENTIA

- Lewy body dementia includes two subtypes: Dementia with Lewy Body (DLB) and Parkinson's Disease Dementia (PDD).
- Lewy bodies are spherical neural inclusions visible in the cortex through staining techniques.
- There are no major differences neuropathologically between DLB and PDD and the classification is still under development. The distinction is mainly on the temporal sequence of appearance of syndromes and in the context of well-established Parkinson's Disease. It is suggested that if dementia arises within 12 months of the extrapyramidal symptoms of Parkinson's Disease being diagnosed then it should be described as DLB. If the dementia develops after 12 months then it is often diagnosed as PDD.
- Patients with Parkinson's Disease have a 24–31 per cent risk of developing PDD.

- DLB often presents with attentional/cognitive fluctuations, visual hallucinations, sleep behaviour disturbances and autonomic dysfunction, whereas in PDD the initial complaints are of movement disorder.
- DLB and PDD are often misdiagnosed and their management is complex.

Further information can be found at the Lewy Body Society: www.lewybody.org

■ FRONTO-TEMPORAL DEMENTIA SYNDROMES (FTDS)

- FTD is sometimes called Pick's disease or frontal lobe dementia.
- FTD is the third most common dementia in the under-65s.
- Around 12 per cent of people diagnosed with dementia under the age of 65 will have FTD.
- FTD is less common in the over-65s.
- FTDs result from neurodegeneration of the frontal and anterior temporal lobes.
- Three main variants are:
  1. Behavioural Variant FTD showing frontal-executive deficits including lack of insight and awareness of consequences of actions;
  2. Progressive Nonfluent Aphasia (PNFA), which presents initially with marked language difficulties particularly in fluency of speech;
  3. Semantic Dementia, where speech fluency is preserved initially but there are marked problems with language comprehension.

- FTDs often present before the age of 65 and are often misdiagnosed.
- Families often experience significant stress and require significant help and support. www.alzheim ers.org.uk/site/scripts/documents_info.php?documen tID=167

■ CREUTZFELDT–JAKOB DISEASE (CJD)

- This is a very rare form of dementia, affecting 1 million people annually worldwide.
- It is a human prion disease characterised by rapid neurodegeneration and spongiform appearance of the brain at post-mortem.
- Symptoms include memory loss, problems with balance and coordination, slurred speech, sight loss, jerky movements and rapid deterioration leading to immobility.
- Different types include:
  - **Variant** – from eating infected meat;
  - **Sporadic** – from a spontaneous mutation of a normal protein;
  - **Iatrogenic** – cross-infection from medical or surgical treatment;
  - **Familial** – rare genetic inheritance in some families.
- Prognosis is poor and death usually occurs within a year from first symptoms (usually from infection).
- There is currently no known cure.
- Treatment is for the relief of pain and comfort.

(www.nhs.uk/Conditions/Creutzfeldt-Jakob-disease/Pages/Introduction.aspx)

■ HUNTINGTON'S DISEASE (HD)

- HD is a progressive neurodegenerative disorder characterised by involuntary movements, behavioural disturbances and dementia.
- HD arises from a genetic mutation on the fourth chromosome and can be an inherited disorder, transmitted via an autosomal dominant pattern, which means each child of a parent with HD has a 50:50 risk of developing it themselves.
- It can occur at any age but most commonly presents in the 40s and 50s, with average life expectancy following diagnosis of 10–20 years.
- Dementia is associated with impaired memory, loss of thought flexibility and mental adjustments. Language function usually remains intact.
- Movement disorders can be helped by medication and exercise.

(www.alzheimer-europe.org/Dementia/Other-forms-of-dementia/Neuro-Degen erative-Diseases/Huntington-s-Disease-HD#fragment-1)

■ DOWN'S SYNDROME DEMENTIA

- People with a learning disability are more likely to develop dementia at a younger age, particularly those with Down's Syndrome.
- One in three people with Down's Syndrome develop Alzheimer's-type dementia by their 50s.

- Early diagnosis is often missed, and may present more with behavioural changes rather than memory loss and the person experiencing the dementia may have difficulty understanding the diagnosis.
- Epilepsy appearing for the first time in later life should trigger an investigation of possible dementia.
- People with a learning disability and dementia require additional help in ensuring their needs for care are met with the changes that dementia brings.

(www.alzheimers.org.uk/site/scripts/documents_info.php?documentID=103
www.bild.org.uk/our-services/books/bestsellers/downs-syndrome-and-dementia/?locale=en)

■ LATE (LIMBIC-PREDOMINANT AGE-RELATED TDP-43 ENCEPHALOPATHY)

- LATE is a newly identified type of dementia.
- LATE occurs due to a build-up of toxic proteins within the brain called TDP-43 in the brain.
- LATE causes damage to the hippocampus and tends to affect memory alone.
- The symptoms of LATE are similar to those of AD.
- Many of those diagnosed with AD may have LATE.
- LATE affects those over 80 more commonly.
- LATE is slower in progression to AD.

Information available at https://academic.oup.com/brain/article/142/6/1503/5481202

■ CHRONIC TRAUMATIC ENCEPHALOPATHY (CTE)

- It is experienced in people with history of contact sports.
- It is a progressive decline of memory and cognition, as well as depression, suicidal behaviour, poor impulse control, aggressiveness, Parkinsonism and eventually dementia.
- It is believed that repetitive brain trauma is responsible for neurodegenerative changes highlighted by accumulations of hyperphosphorylated tau and TDP-43 proteins.
- These symptoms often begin years or even decades after the last brain trauma or end of active athletic involvement.
- Currently, CTE can only be diagnosed after death.

More information at www.nhs.uk/conditions/chronic-trauma tic-encephalopathy/

■ ALCOHOL-RELATED BRAIN DAMAGE (ARBD)

- Alcohol-related brain damage (ARBD) or alcohol-related brain injury (ARBI) (www.alzheimers.org.uk) is a brain disorder caused by excessive drinking over years, causing damage to nerve cells, damage to vessels and lack of thiamine.
- Unlike dementia progression can be halted and in some cases reversed with treatment and abstinence.
- Around 10 per cent of those with dementia will have ARBD.

- There are several specific types of ARBD. The two most common types are:
  1. alcohol-related 'dementia' caused from damage of excessive drinking over a period of time;
  2. Wernicke–Korsakoff syndrome (Korsakoff Syndrome) caused specifically by the lack of thiamine normally through drinking over a period of time. Wernicke–Korsakoff syndrome has two stages. Firstly, there will be intense inflammation (swelling) of their brain. known as 'Wernicke's encephalopathy'. If not treated as an emergency this can lead to long term brain damage and 'Korsakoff's syndrome' or possibly death.
- Around 40 per cent of alcoholics experience mild cognitive impairment due to cerebral shrinkage, more pronounced in older people and more apparent in the frontal lobe.
- Typically people present with Korsakoff's aged 45–65, but it also occurs in people who are younger and older.
- It is more common in men than women.
- In Korsakoff's Syndrome, memory is severely affected but other cognitive functions can appear relatively intact. Confabulation (making up a convincing story to fill in memory gaps) is common.
- The progress of Korsakoff's Syndrome can be halted if the person abstains from alcohol and has a healthy diet with vitamin supplements. Without these lifestyle changes, the damage continues to progress.

- Korsakoff's Syndrome is often but not always preceded by Wernicke's Encephalopathy, and is therefore also known as Wernicke–Korsakoff syndrome.
- Alcohol-related dementia includes substantial damage to the cerebral cortex. Korsakoff's can co-exist with other dementias.

(www.alzheimers.org.uk/site/scripts/documents_info.php?documentID=98)

■ POST-DIAGNOSTIC SUPPORT

Useful resources for information in relation to post-diagnosis support include:

- NICE quick guide for people with dementia and their families at: www.nice.org.uk/about/nice-communities/social-care/quick-guides/dementia-discussing-and-planning-support-after-diagnosis
- Dementia UK checklist at: www.dementiauk.org/get-support/diagnosis-and-next-steps/after-a-diagnosis-of-dementia-next-steps-checklist/
- NHS dementia guide at: www.nhs.uk/conditions/dementia/help-and-support/
- UK government policy joint declaration paper at: www.gov.uk/government/publications/dementia-post-diagnostic-care-and-support/dementia-post-diagnostic-care-and-support

4   Pharmacological Treatments for Dementia

- Currently there is no treatment that can convincingly alter the course of the underlying disease processes of dementia.
- Pharmacological treatments can improve mental performance.
- NICE guidelines are provided, and these are subject to change as new drugs and research become available. See http://guidance.nice.org.uk for the latest information.

■ CHOLINESTERASE INHIBITORS

- Donepezil (Aricept), Rivastigmine (Exelon) and Galantamine (Reminyl) work by improving the communication between brain cells that are weakened by Alzheimer's Disease or Lewy Body dementia.
- In Alzheimer's Disease 40–70 per cent of patients show some benefit (Alzheimer's Society 2021).
- In Lewy Body dementia the benefit can be more noticeable, with improved concentration and a decrease in visual hallucinations.

■ MEMANTINE

- Memantine (Ebixa) works by blocking the effects of pathologically elevated toxic levels of glutamate.
- There is still some debate about the usefulness of Memantine and, at the time of going to press, NICE (2018) only recommends this for people who are

DOI: 10.4324/9781003269946-4

intolerant to cholinesterase inhibitors, or where there are contraindications for their use.

For the prescription of these drugs NICE also requires that:

- For people who are not taking an AChE inhibitor or Memantine, prescribers should only start treatment with these on the advice of a clinician who has the necessary knowledge and skills. This could include:
  - secondary care medical specialists such as psychiatrists, geriatricians and neurologists
  - other healthcare professionals (such as GPs, nurse consultants and advanced nurse practitioners), if they have specialist expertise in diagnosing and treating Alzheimer's Disease.
- AChE inhibitors, in people with Alzheimer's Disease, should not be stopped because of disease severity alone.
- Ensure that local arrangements for prescribing, supply and treatment review follow the NICE guideline on medicines optimisation.
- A person on the treatment is reviewed by a specialist (but not necessarily a doctor) every six months.

5   Families as Partners in Care

- Family carers are critical to the quality of life of those they support.
- The vast majority of care for people living with dementia is undertaken by families. Many family care-givers report high levels of burden, stress, depressive symptoms and social isolation.
- There can be many reasons for becoming a care-giver, some of which are love, duty, guilt, expectation and societal pressure.
- Daily challenges include direct supervision and communication, managing risk and coping with the changing relationship as the person's cognitive abilities change.
- 'Carer burden' is a term that has previously been used to describe the extent to which family care-givers perceive that their emotional or physical health, social life and financial status suffer as a result of caring for their relative.
- Although caring can be rewarding, for a large percentage of people it can also bring many challenges.
- Understanding the rewards and challenges faced by care-givers is critical to enable appropriate support to be offered.
- The past and current relationship quality appears to have an impact on family care-givers' well-being. When there have been poor-quality relationship problems prior to the

DOI: 10.4324/9781003269946-5

onset of the dementia then there are likely to be greater feelings of burden as the dementia progresses.

- The reason for undertaking the role can have a direct impact upon feelings of burden.
- The level of dependency, alongside the level of behavioural problems, influences the family care-giver's perceptions of relationship quality.
- Those who are highly dependent and have a higher number of distressed behaviours are more likely to have family care-givers who report higher levels of burden.
- Hospital admissions are a particularly stressful time for families, often coming at the end of a period of high stress marked by sleepless nights and high anxiety.
- Families react to this stress in different ways. Some need to take a complete break. Others may feel very reluctant to leave their dependent relative in the care of others.
- It is important to adopt a non-judgemental approach in regard to the level of involvement that families have in care.
- Families need to be included as partners in care.
- Families need to be recognised as significant in telling the story and providing a history of the problems that the patient is presenting with.
- Many hospitals use a system of gathering information from families on admission. This information can then be used to form the basis of the care plan and assist with helping the patient feel settled. An example of this is 'This is me', which can be downloaded from: www.alzheimers. org.uk/get-support/publications-factsheets/this-is-me

- Some families will be able to write this information down and will be pleased to do so. Others will need more help and it might be necessary to use such a document to build up knowledge about the person over the first few days following admission.
- The sooner the care team have this information, however, the easier it will be to provide person-centred care for the patient, which will minimise distress and ensure that the skills the patient has are not lost because of being in hospital.

■ USEFUL WEBSITES FOR FAMILY CARERS

- Admiral Nurses: www.dementiauk.org/what-we-do/admiral-nurses
- Alzheimer's Disease International: www.alzint.org/about/
- Alzheimer Scotland: www.alzscot.org/
- Alzheimer's Society: www.alzheimers.org.uk/Caring_for_someone_with_dementia/
- Carers UK: www.carersuk.org
- Citizens Advice Bureau: www.citizensadvice.org.uk
- Cross Roads and Princess Royal Trust (now Carers Trust): www.carers.org.uk
- Dementia UK: www.dementiauk.org
- The Relatives and Residents Association: www.relres.org/

6   Capacity

Dementia can affect cognitive abilities associated with decision making. Legislation, Department of Health (DoH) and NICE guidelines address this issue, providing practical guidance for healthcare professionals:

- Reference guide to consent for examination or treatment, 2nd edition, 2009: www.dh.gov.uk/en/Publicationsandsta tistics/Publications/PublicationsPolicyAndGuidance/DH_ 103643
- Mental Capacity Act 2005: www.gov.uk/government/publi cations/mental-capacity-act-code-of-practice
- Code of Practice, 2015: www.gov.uk/government/publi cations/code-of-practice-mental-health-act-1983

■   MENTAL CAPACITY ACT (MCA)

- The MCA sets out a statutory framework for making decisions on behalf of people who lack capacity to make decisions for themselves.
- When followed correctly, it provides protection from liability for treatment decisions made by healthcare staff under the Act.
- The framework acknowledges that an individual's capacity to make a decision can vary over time, according to the decision that needs to be made and depending on the person's circumstances. Therefore, assessing a person's capacity must be both time- and decisions-specific.

DOI: 10.4324/9781003269946-6

- A person may lack the capacity to make a complex decision (such as moving into residential care) but that does not mean that they cannot be involved with aspects of that decision (such as the location) or with other, less complex decisions (such as what time to get up).

The MCA Code of Practice provides detailed guidance on how to apply the MCA in practice. The **five core principles** of the MCA must guide staff actions:

1 A person must be assumed to have capacity unless it is established that they lack capacity.
2 A person should not be treated as unable to make a decision unless all practicable steps have been taken to help them make a decision.
3 A person is not to be treated as unable to make a decision merely because they make an unwise decision.
4 An act done, or a decision made, on behalf of a person who lacks capacity must be done or made in their best interests.
5 Before an act done, or a decision made, regard must be had to whether the purpose for which it is needed can be as effectively achieved in a way that is less restrictive of the person's rights and freedom of action.

■ ASSESSING CAPACITY

- Staff must be able to demonstrate 'reasonable belief' that a person lacks capacity to make a particular decision, in order to lawfully act on their behalf.

- This is not simply about whether the person has dementia, but about evidencing the effect that the dementia may have on the person's decision-making abilities.
- The MCA outlines a 'two-stage test' of capacity, both parts of which are equally important:
  1 Does the person have an impairment of, or disturbance in, the functioning of their mind or brain (such as a dementia)?
  2 If so, is the impairment or disturbance sufficient enough to cause the person to be unable to make the particular decision at the relevant time?

There are four key issues that help determine whether a person's dementia may be impairing their ability to make a decision:

1 Can the person **understand** information relevant to the decision, including understanding the likely consequences of making, or not making, the decision?
2 Can they **retain** this information for long enough to make the decision?
3 Can they **use and weigh** the information to arrive at a choice?
4 Can they **communicate** their decision in any way?

■ BEST INTERESTS DECISION MAKING

- If a person is unable to make a particular decision for themselves, decisions must be made in the person's best interests.

- The following provides guidance on best interests decision making: www.nice.org.uk/guidance/ng108/chapter/recommendations

Best interests decision making must:
- not be discriminatory (not based solely on the person's age, appearance or behaviour);
- involve the person as much as possible;
- have regard for the person's past and present wishes, feelings and beliefs;
- consider the likelihood of the person regaining capacity;
- consult with others who know the person well, including family, friends, care staff and professionals;
- in relation to life-sustaining treatment, not be motivated by a desire to bring about the person's death.

If the person has no family or friends who can speak for them (or there are safeguarding concerns regarding those individuals) and serious medical treatment decisions have to be made, the person must be supported by an Independent Mental Capacity Advocate (IMCA) to advocate on their behalf.

■ LEAST RESTRICTIVE ACTIONS AND DEPRIVATION OF LIBERTY

- Best interests decisions must always be carried out in a way that is **least restrictive** of the person's rights and freedoms. This means that restriction or restraint of a person can only be lawfully used when it is proportional to the likelihood and seriousness of potential harm to the person.

- Restriction or restraint includes not only physical restraint but also measures such as chemical restraint (sedation), benign force (deception) and environmental restraint (locked doors/puzzle locks).
- If a person is judged to lack capacity and the best interest decision made for that person requires the use of restriction or restraint, then strict guidelines must be followed. In the event that the restriction or restraint required could constitute a deprivation of the person's liberty, then the hospital, NHS trust or care home (the 'Managing Authority') **must** apply for an authorisation through the Deprivation of Liberty Safeguards (DoLS) process in order to carry out the action lawfully.
- Authorisations should be sought before the action is taken.
- In emergency situations a managing authority may grant itself an 'urgent authorisation' but it must be simultaneously applied for with 'standard authorisation' through the DoLS process.
- There is no standard definition of what constitutes a deprivation of liberty, because it depends on the impact of the measure/s on the individual. However, examples of possible deprivations of liberty include:
  - use of force or sedation to admit a person or prevent them from leaving;
  - deceiving a person into cooperating (particularly in relation to admittance);

- objection by a person's relatives/carers to them being admitted or remaining in the setting;
- persistent and purposeful attempts by a person to leave that are prevented by force or a locked door (or an immobile person asking to leave persistently and purposefully);
- organising a person's care in such a way that severely restricts what they can do in other ways (e.g. using furniture from which they cannot get up).
- Guidelines for use of DoLS are available in the DoLS Code of Practice, found at: www.dh.gov.uk.
- Guidance on what may constitute a deprivation of liberty and further details about the DoLS process are available from the Alzheimer's Society: www.alzheimers. org.uk/site/scripts/documents_info.php?document ID=1327

■ MCA PROVISIONS

- When an individual lacks capacity in regard to a certain decision, there are a number of provisions created by the MCA that may place responsibility for decision making with a certain individual. These are as follows (in order of procedure):
  1. a relevant **Advance Decision**;
  2. a valid **Lasting Power of Attorney** (LPA);
  3. a **Deputy** appointed by the Court of Protection.
- Healthcare professionals should ensure that none of these applies before undertaking decision making themselves.

■ ADVANCE CARE PLANNING

- Making an advance decision needs to be considered from as early a point as possible when the person still has capacity to be involved. As dementia progresses the window of opportunity to complete these will shrink.
- There are three parts to advance care planning:
  - making statements about future needs and wishes;
  - making Advance Decisions to Refuse Treatment;
  - making a Lasting Power of Attorney.

All three are not required and can be completed at different times.

■ STATEMENTS ABOUT FUTURE NEEDS AND WISHES

- These consist of a written statement of a person's treatment preferences, which a healthcare professional should take into account when considering best interests. They are sometimes called 'advance statements'.
- They can cover care, support, treatment and preferred place of care.
- They don't necessarily need to be written down, it is best to do this.
- It is also important to decide the best place to keep these statements so relevant people have access to these.
- They are not legally binding but can assist with a best interests decision that can then be made that meant the wishes of the person with dementia had not been followed. Best interests decisions must take into account

the person's views and wishes as much as possible –
including those made in advance.

■ ADVANCE DECISIONS TO REFUSE TREATMENT

- An advance decision is a legally binding written
  statement refusing certain life-sustaining treatment. It is
  distinct from a written statement of a person's treatment
  preferences.
- In terms of medical decisions, doctors must comply with
  advance decisions to refuse life-sustaining treatment
  unless it is found that the person lacked capacity
  at the time the advance decision was made, or if new
  treatments have been developed that may have
  affected the person's advance decision had they known
  about them at the time they made it.

The advance decision:

- must specify the life-sustaining treatment that is to be
  refused;
- should set out the circumstances in which the refusal
  will apply;
- can be expressed in medical or lay terms;
- will only apply when the person making it has lost
  capacity;
- can be altered or withdrawn at any time while the person
  making it has capacity;
- need not be in writing *unless* it is about necessary life-
  sustaining treatment;

- must be in writing, signed and witnessed and must include a statement that the decision is to apply even if life is at risk – if it relates to refusing life-sustaining treatment;
- has the same status as when a person with capacity refuses treatment (as long as it is valid and applicable).

■ IS THE DECISION VALID?

An advance decision is **not valid** if:

- it has been withdrawn;
- the person has acted in a way that is clearly inconsistent with the advance decision.

■ IS THE DECISION APPLICABLE?

An advance decision is **applicable** if:

- it clearly refers to the treatment in question;
- the circumstances are the same as set out in the advance decision;
- there are no reasonable grounds for believing that circumstances have changed that would have affected the advance decision.

More information can be found at: www.scie.org.uk/dementia/supporting-people-with-dementia/decisions/advance-care-planning.asp

■ LASTING POWER OF ATTORNEY (LPA)

- A person can appoint another named person to have the authority to make decisions on their behalf should they lack capacity to make decisions for themselves at some point in the future.
- The person receiving the power of attorney is called the 'donee' or 'attorney', and the person granting it is called the donor.
- An LPA can be made for 'personal welfare/healthcare' and/or for 'finance/property' decisions (see below).
- Decisions made using LPA must be in the person's best interests.
- Serious concerns relating to decisions taken under LPA can be referred to the Court of Protection.

More information can be found at: www.alzheimers.org.uk/get-support/legal-financial/lasting-power-attorney

■ PERSONAL WELFARE/HEALTHCARE LPA

- It can only be used when the person has lost capacity.
- It can be used to make decisions about all or specified personal welfare/healthcare matters (depending on what the donor has specified).
- If LPA expressly says so, they can give the attorney authority to give/refuse consent to life-sustaining treatment.

■ FINANCIAL AND PROPERTY LPA

- LPA financial agreements can take effect before the donor has lost mental capacity.
- It can be used to make decisions about all or specified matters concerning property and affairs (depending on what the donor has specified).

■ THE COURT OF PROTECTION AND DEPUTIES

The Court of Protection has the power to:
- make declarations about a person's capacity or the lawfulness of a particular act (e.g. major medical treatment);
- make single decisions (e.g. selling a property or deciding where someone should live);
- appoint a 'deputy' who has ongoing authority to make decisions;
- decide whether an LPA is valid;
- remove an attorney who is not acting in the donor's best interests.

The Court process will be a last resort and most people need permission to apply.

■ ETHICAL DECISION MAKING

The Nuffield Council on Bioethics (2009) has developed six components in relation to ethical issues for people with dementia:
1 care-based approach to ethical decisions;
2 a belief about the nature of dementia;

3 a belief about quality of life for the person with dementia;
4 the importance of promoting the interests of both the person with dementia and those who care for them;
5 the requirement to act in accordance with solidarity;
6 recognising personhood, identity and value.

7 Pain Assessment and Management

- Pain assessment and management in patients with dementia is often overlooked.
- If a person with dementia appears agitated, irritable or is shouting out it may be that they are unable to communicate directly about an underlying painful condition.
- Looking out for signs of pain and assessing for conditions that might cause pain, such as arthritis or bad teeth, can sometimes provide an answer. Appropriate use of simple analgesia may be all that is needed.
- Research suggests that even though older patients are more likely to be in pain than younger patients, they receive less pain relief, while patients with dementia receive even less pain management than older people who are not cognitively impaired.

■ PAIN ASSESSMENT TOOLS FOR PEOPLE WITH DEMENTIA

Most regular pain assessment tools rely on verbal reports, as follows:

- Self-reporting (gold standard): https://dontforgetthebubbles.com/self-report-pain-scales/
- Visual Analogue Scale (VAS): www.blackwellpublishing.com/specialarticles/jcn_10_706.pdf
- Verbal Rating Scales (VRS), e.g. http://pain.about.com/od/testingdiagnosis/ig/pain-scales/McGill-Pain-Scale.htm

DOI: 10.4324/9781003269946-7

- Numeric Rating Scales (NRS), e.g. http://pain.about.com/od/testingdiagnosis/ig/pain-scales/McGill-Pain-Scale.htm

In dementia, pain assessment tools that use non-verbal signs are required when the person can no longer verbally communicate their pain, including:
- The Abbey Pain Scale: www.wales.nhs.uk/sitesplus/documents/862/foi-286f-13.pdf
- Non-Communicative Patient's Pain Assessment Instrument (NOPPAIN): https://bcpsqc.ca/wp-content/uploads/2018/11/NOPPAIN.pdf
- Disability Distress Assessment Tool (DisDAT): www.disdat.co.uk/
- DOLOPLUS-2 (Behavioural pain assessment in the elderly): https://prc.coh.org/PainNOA/Doloplus%202_Tool.pdf

■ NON-VERBAL PAIN INDICATORS

Non-verbal pain indicators include:
- vocalisation (groaning, crying, calling out);
- facial expressions (frowning, grimacing);
- body language (rocking, guarding, withdrawing, massaging area);
- behaviour/activity change (confusion, withdrawal, inability to stay still, refusing to eat);
- physiological indicators (blood pressure, flushing, perspiring, pulse);
- timing, duration, aggravating factors.

Physiological signs and symptoms for the person in pain may include:
- acute/high-intensity pain (e.g. blood pressure, heart rate);
- higher threshold for autonomic activity;
- low-intensity pain, which induces smaller autonomic responses, i.e. autonomic responses in non-communicative patients may indicate high-level pain intensity. (Note: low autonomic responses to pain do not reflect absence of pain.)

■ CARING FOR A PERSON WITH DEMENTIA WHO IS IN PAIN

- Identify the severity and type of pain using the appropriate assessment tool.
- If a person can articulate pain use a verbal rating scale
- If a person cannot articulate pain use an observational tool.
- Seek to understand whether there has been a change from the person's normal behaviour in order to note any changes that might indicate pain.
- Get a comprehensive history from carers/family/advocate to find out how the person reacts when pain is present.
- Maintain a familiar and comfortable environment.
- Remember that pain is assumed when a diagnosis that is painful in patients without dementia is given, even though the person with dementia may not be able to express themselves.

- Give analgesics if there is any sign or diagnosis that in normal circumstances would result in someone expressing they have pain.
- Use an assessment tool to monitor improvements or decline.

8   Nutrition and Hydration

Nutrition and hydration are important aspects of caring for people with dementia, who are at high risk of being malnourished (Age Concern 2006, 2010). There are a number of factors that can result in someone living with dementia becoming malnourished or dehydrated, such as:

- memory problems (forgetting to eat or thinking that they have already eaten);
- apraxia (loss of ability to use common objects, such as cutlery);
- change in lifestyle, including loss of independence and eating habits;
- problems with swallowing (dysphagia);
- changing nutritional needs;
- decreased sensory abilities in taste, smell, hearing and sight;
- physical impairments;
- poor oral health;
- digestive problems;
- medications that affect appetite or cause a dry mouth;
- socioeconomic factors that influence the availability of preferred foods;
- cultural and religious beliefs not being recognised;
- poor preparation of food;
- physical environment not conducive to eating well.

DOI: 10.4324/9781003269946-8

■ ASSESSMENT OF NUTRITIONAL NEEDS

- Assessment should include how, where, when and with whom the person associates food and eating.
- At all times the person's dignity and personhood should be maintained through familiar rituals and eating habits.
- Cognitive impairments should be taken into consideration, such as orientation, short-term recall, visuo-spatial perception, reasoning, planning and communication skills.
- Common assessment tools for assessment of a person's nutritional state include:
  1 Malnutrition Universal Screening Tool (MUST): www. bapen.org.uk/pdfs/must/must_full.pdf
  2 Edinburgh Feeding Evaluation in Dementia (EdFED) (Watson et al. 2001) for assessment of feeding difficulty.

At the later stages, people with dementia may need a lot of help with eating and drinking.

- If the person spits food out, leaves their mouth open when food is placed in it or refuses food it is necessary to assess the underlying reasons for this. This can be due to physiological reasons, such as mouth or throat pain, cognitive problems to do with dysphagia or mood disorders, such as depression.
- This can cause distress for the family and carers and it is important to take it seriously.

■ WEIGHT LOSS

Weight loss can result from:

- increased activity with pacing and moving or due to changes within the hypothalamus, which regulates food intake and metabolic rate;
- atrophy of the mesial temporal cortex, which may affect the eating behaviour, memory and behaviour;
- cognitive impairments, including thinking have just eaten or being worried about not liking food, worries over spilling or making a mess, worries about choking, problems with swallowing and chewing;
- reduction in the taste sensation so that food appears bland and unappetising.

■ WEIGHT GAIN

Weight gain can result from:

- increased static lifestyle, either from lack of opportunity to exercise or decreased motivation because of low mood;
- physical pain leading to decreased activity levels;
- cognitive impairments, such as a person thinking they have not eaten when in fact they have, which can result in overeating and poor monitoring of intake.

■ HELPING A PERSON WITH DEMENTIA TO EAT

Mealtimes should strive to:

- use familiar cooking smells to whet the appetite;
- be familiar and homelike;

- be within a calm environment;
- use clear place settings (e.g. high contrast between crockery and table);
- use attractive but uncluttered table space;
- use appropriate eating implements for the person's culture;
- use appropriate eating implements for the level of cognitive impairment (e.g. the person may not be able to use a knife and fork but may happily eat with a spoon);
- provide food that can easily be picked up for people who are happier feeding themselves with their fingers;
- utilise adequate lighting so people can see what they are eating;
- ensure food looks appetising;
- provide a choice of food presented at meal times (orders from previous day will often be forgotten);
- maintain normal eating patterns in terms of timing and types of food and drink;
- be a social event where appropriate.

When assisting with eating:
- Introduce yourself and explain that you are going to help the person to eat or drink.
- Achieve eye contact where possible, position yourself on a level with the person being helped.
- Help the person to put their hand over yours – this may help them feel more in control of the speed of the eating.
- Touch spoon to lips.

- Be aware not to overload spoon and give the person enough time to swallow.
- Provide ongoing verbal cueing (e.g. tell the person what is happening).
- Reposition yourself on a different side or to the front if you are not getting a response.
- Encourage eating with other people, which may cue in eating behaviour.

■ TUBE/ENTERAL FEEDING

- There is no evidence to support that tube feeding results in any extension of life, improvement in nutritional outcomes, reduction in the incidence of leg ulcers or improvement in the quality of life in people in the latter stages of dementia (Candy et al. 2009).
- Tube feeding can result in an increase in the complications relating to nutrition and caring for people with advanced dementia.

9   Dementia-Friendly Environments

- Environments that are designed specifically for people with dementia can reduce the incidence of agitation and challenging behaviours, encourage meaningful activities, increase feelings of well-being, decrease falls and accidents and improve continence and mobility. See The Kings Fund, Environments of care for people with dementia: www.kingsfund.org.uk/current_projects/enhancing_the_healing_environment/
- Simple changes can improve the quality of care considerably:
  - Ensure people have access to glasses, hearing aid, walking aid if used.
  - Ensure their path is free of hazards/barriers if they want to walk to the toilet or to get assistance.
  - Use clear signage and personal objects to orientate people.
  - Provide clear notices, clocks and calendars to aid orientation.
  - Ensure that help and assistance are easy to find. Ensure toilet signs are clear.
  - Have adequate storage to put hazardous and confusing objects out of sight.
  - Have lots of items that are interesting and safe to handle.
  - Have adequate lighting. People who are very old need light that is twice as bright as middle-aged people.
  - Use lots of natural light rather than artificial light.

DOI: 10.4324/9781003269946-9

- Be aware the glare and shadows may create perceptual problems and misunderstandings for people with cognitive visual-spatial perceptual impairments.
- Avoid sudden contrasts on flooring and shiny floors, which may be perceived as hazardous.
- Avoid patterns on floors – they may be perceived as clutter or objects.
- Cut out extraneous and sudden unexpected noise.
- Nature and access to fresh air and greenery are important in promoting well-being.

10 Behavioural and Psychological Symptoms of Dementia (BPSD)

- BPSD is a way of describing many of the common non-cognitive problems that cause difficulties for people as dementia progresses. Guidance can be found on the International Psychogeriatric Association website: www.ipa-online.org/publications/guides-to-bpsd
- BPSD is formally assessed using the Neuropsychiatric Inventory (www.cgakit.com/p-3-npi) and includes:
  - delusions;
  - hallucinations;
  - agitation;
  - depressed mood;
  - anxiety;
  - apathy;
  - irritability;
  - euphoria;
  - disinhibition;
  - aberrant motor behaviour;
  - night-time behaviour disturbances;
  - appetite and eating abnormalities.
- The majority of people with dementia will experience BPSD at some point.
- They are often the sorts of problems for which anti-psychotic medication is prescribed, but this can have many undesirable side-effects.

DOI: 10.4324/9781003269946-10

- The first task is to understand why the symptom is occurring and to identify ways of ameliorating it that does not involve anti-psychotic medication.
- Guidelines and assessment tools are free to download at www.alzheimers.org.uk/site/scripts/download_info.php?downloadID=609
- Each type of BPSD may be caused by a multiplicity of different causes.
- Where BPSD is not ameliorated by good-quality person-centred care, and the impact of any acute confusional state has been ruled out, then a referral may be required to specialist psychiatric or psychological services to undertake specific, functional, analysis-based interventions.

■ GET A CLEAR DESCRIPTION OF THE BEHAVIOUR

The first task is to be very clear on what the behaviour or psychological symptom is. Using general terms, such as aggression or disinhibition, is not useful in helping to understand the problem.

Ask yourself the following:

- What is the patient doing or saying?
- What is the emotional state of the patient?
- Who does this happen with?
- When does it happen?
- Where does it happen?
- How long has this been going on?
- What are the possible triggers?
- What is the frequency and duration?

It is also useful to identify who the behaviour is distressing, because this will impact on the strategy or strategies required. Is it …

- the person with dementia themselves?
- the family members?
- other patients on the ward or residents in the home?
- the staff?

■ NEURO-PSYCHOLOGICAL FACTORS

- The type of neurological damage may be significant. For example, if the patient has damage in their visual cortex it may mean that they see things that are not there (hallucinations).
- Environmental changes can help here to make the hallucinations less likely; changing lighting can help.
- Assistive technologies can help to orientate people or keep them safe.
- Cognitive Stimulation Therapy (CST) helps cognition, mood and feelings of well-being in mild to moderate dementia: www.cstdementia.com
- Cognitive prompts and repeated practice can help to establish new routines and help with everyday tasks.

■ LIFE STORY FACTORS

- Incidents in the person's past may trigger a negative reaction. For example, if the patient had wartime experiences where they were mistreated in a hospital-like environment it may trigger an aggressive reaction when they are cared for by people in uniform.

- Staff understand the person with dementia better if they know their life story.
- Knowing something about the person's life story will enable more positive memories to be prompted.
- Recalling the happy or proud moments from the past plays to the person's strengths. It is an enjoyable shared activity for family members.
- Objects, photos, music and dance stimulate memories. Such activities help people to maintain a sense of identity.
- More information on life stories can be found at www. lifestorynetwork.org.uk

■ PHYSICAL HEALTH (SEE ALSO CHAPTER 7, 'PAIN ASSESSMENT AND MANAGEMENT')

- Untreated physical health problems cause restlessness or agitation or pain.
- Physical exercise helps mood, cognition, agitation and sleep problems. Keep a regular routine.
- Pain is very under-recognised and under-treated in people with dementia.
- People with dementia are poor at reporting symptoms of illness or pain. Any noticeable sudden increase in confusion needs investigating.

■ QUALITY OF CARE

- Poor-quality care and communication can produce an emotional reaction that is then misinterpreted as a behavioural problem.

- Excessive sleepiness may occur because people are bored or under-stimulated.
- General person-centred care minimises the escalation of problems into BPSD.
- People with dementia have a better mood and quality of life if they are cared for by staff who communicate well.
- Aromatherapy, massage, multisensory stimulation and music may all be helpful to some people to instil a feeling of calm.
- For more evidence-based ideas see: www.alzheimers. org.uk/get-involved/engagement-participation/engagem ent-projects-personal-stories/facing-it-together-fit-group and www.carefitforvips.co.uk

■ DEPRESSION

- People with dementia are more likely to experience depression.
- This might be as a direct result of dementia affecting the mood centre of the brain or due to the changes in coping skills that often accompany dementia.
- The best response to depression is an individual one aimed at improving quality of life rather than looking to medication.
- If depression is very persistent, especially when it continues for a long time, or if there are 'biological symptoms' such as poor appetite or a tendency to wake early, anti-depressants can be helpful.

- There is rarely any benefit for the first two weeks of anti-depressant therapy and it may take a few more weeks after that for the full improvement to develop.
- There are several different classes of anti-depressant drug, with different effects and side-effects. The older variety, known as tricyclics (e.g. Amitriptyline), are best avoided in older people as they have more side-effects, including making memory worse.

■ ANTI-PSYCHOTIC DRUGS

- Anti-psychotics were developed for treating severe mental illness such as schizophrenia and most have very little evidence to support their use in dementia.
- Examples of such drugs include: atypical anti-psychotics (e.g. Risperidone, Amisulpride, Quetiapine); typical anti-psychotics (e.g. Haloperidol); benzodiazepines (e.g. Diazepam and Lorazepam); and anti-depressants with sedating properties (e.g. Trazodone).
- Adverse effects of anti-psychotics include:
  - Parkinsonism;
  - falls;
  - dehydration;
  - chest infection/pneumonia;
  - ankle oedema;
  - DVT/PE;
  - cardiac arrhythmia;
  - stroke;
  - over-sedation.

- Anti-psychotic medication should not be used in patients with Lewy Body dementia unless there is expert supervision.
- Many BPSDs decrease significantly over time without drug treatment and the advice is usually to hold off prescribing medication for a period of four weeks to assess other non-drug interventions first (Alzheimer's Society 2011).
- Drug treatment may continue to have a small part to play in helping people with dementia with these distressing states, but only as part of a wider understanding of the problem and a broader approach to alleviating distress (Sturdy et al. 2012).

■ ANTI-PSYCHOTIC PRESCRIBING FOR PATIENTS WITH DELIRIUM

- According to the current NICE guidelines CG 103 (2010, updated 2019), medication should only be given in delirium if the person is distressed, or considered at risk to self and/or others, and where de-escalation techniques have proved ineffective.

Please refer to most recent NICE guidelines:
- National Prescribing Centre, now part of NICE: www.nice.org.uk/mpc
- NICE guidelines on 'Supporting people with dementia and their carers in health and social care': www.nice.org.uk/guidance/cg42

- The Department of Health's 'Antipsychotics: initiative to reduce prescribing to older people with dementia': www.gov.uk/drug-safety-update/antipsychotics-initiative-to-reduce-prescribing-to-older-people-with-dementia

11 Acute Confusional States (Delirium) and Dementia

- When someone has the label of dementia, there is a risk that any increase in confused behaviour is attributed to the dementia.
- People with dementia are much more susceptible to acute confusional states and delirium arising from physical health problems, such as urinary or chest infections, constipation, hormonal imbalances, dehydration, malnutrition, over-medication and sedation.
- Many people with dementia will not be able to give an accurate account of their symptoms because of their memory problems. For example, if a person with dementia is unable to remember that they have been experiencing chest pains, they are unlikely to report symptoms.
- Healthcare staff need to be extra-attentive to changes in physical health status that may not be reported by the patient directly.

■ WHAT IS DELIRIUM?

- Acute confusional state, or delirium, is defined as a disturbed consciousness, cognitive function or perception (NICE 2010, updated 2019).
- It is characterised by an acute onset and often presents as noticeable fluctuations in behaviour.
- It is caused by pathophysiology but presents as a disorder of cognition (Scofield 2008).

DOI: 10.4324/9781003269946-11

- Taking a medical history from the patient or carer will usually identify that this confusional state is of recent origin. It is also totally reversible with treatment.

■ GENERAL SYMPTOMS

- change in behaviour;
- slow responses;
- visual or auditory hallucinations;
- reduced mobility;
- changes in appetite;
- sleep disturbances;
- changes in mood and cooperation;
- increased difficulty communicating.

Delirium can present as hypoactive or hyperactive; however, a person can also present with a mixed type, which is more difficult to recognise.

■ RISK FACTORS

- dementia;
- any severe illness;

Table 11.1 Type of delirium and possible symptoms

TYPE	POSSIBLE SYMPTOMS
Hypoactive	Withdrawn, quiet, sleepy
Hyperactive	Heightened arousal, restless, agitated, aggressive

- fractured hip;
- anaesthetic;
- high alcohol intake;
- dehydration;
- constipation;
- acute infections;
- polypharmacy;
- other drugs.

■ COMPLICATIONS

- Longer hospital stays resulting in:
    - more hospital-acquired complications;
    - pressure sores;
    - falls;
    - more likely to be admitted to long-term care;
    - more likely to die.

■ TREATMENT

- Assess cause(s) of delirium.
- Check for and treat underlying infection.
- Check for hypoxia and give oxygen if necessary.
- Check for and treat constipation.
- Rehydrate the patient.
- Address any pain.
- Address poor nutrition.
- Address sensory impairment.
- Promote good sleep patterns and sleep hygiene.
- Attend to mobilisation.
- Recognise the person may be acting out of character.

- Maintain the person's dignity.
- Provide regular orientation and reassurance.
- Use information about the person's identity to reinforce the patient's perceptions of who they are and provide anchors into the here and now.
- Encourage contact with family and friends where possible but recognise that changes in behaviour may be difficult for some family members.
- Reassure family and friends that the increased confusion and changes in behaviour are temporary.

12 End-of-Life Care

- Dementia is the leading cause of death in the UK accounting for 12.7 per cent of all deaths (Office for National Statistics 2020).
- Dementia is the leading cause of death for females and the second for males in the UK (Office for National Statistics 2020).
- The principles of palliative care are appropriate at any time for the person with dementia and their family and carers.
- As the person with dementia's condition progresses, their need for greater physical care and accommodation for behavioural changes will also increase.
- The official position paper of the European Association for Palliative Care (EAPC Onlus) defines palliative care in dementia by describing its core domains and by defining optimal care. It presents a set of recommendations for all those who provide palliative care to people with dementia (van der Steen et al. 2014).
- The National Council for Palliative Care (2006) offers guidance on the needs of people with dementia at the end of their lives.
- NICE (2015) guideline covers the clinical care of adults including those with dementia who are dying during the last two to three days of life. It aims to improve end-of-life care for people in their last days of life by communicating respectfully and involving them, and the people important to them, in decisions and by

DOI: 10.4324/9781003269946-12

maintaining their comfort and dignity and supporting them (www.nice.org.uk/guidance/ng31).

- The National Institute for Health and Clinical Excellence, in collaboration with the Social Care Institute for Excellence (NICE-SCIE 2007), has identified key principles for palliative care and dementia as a benchmark for care planning and implementation. These include that dementia sufferers should live and die with dignity in a place of their choice; also, that the emphasis is on the quality of life, and carers should be supported throughout.

■ USEFUL RESOURCES

- Leadership Alliance for the Care of Dying People (2014). One chance to get it right. London: Leadership Alliance for the Care of Dying People: https://assets.publishing. service.gov.uk/government/uploads/system/uploads/atta chment_data/file/323188/One_chance_to_get_it_right. pdf and
- Marie Curie web resource – caring for someone with dementia towards end of life www.mariecurie.org.uk/ professionals/palliative-care-knowledge-zone/condition-specific-short-guides/dementia
- NHS Choices website – dementia and end of life planning: www.nhs.uk/conditions/dementia/palliat ive-care/
- Department of Health End of Life Care Programme: www. endoflifecareforadults.nhs.uk www.dyingmatters.org/ page/people-dementia

- Gold Standards Framework (GSF): www.goldstandardsframework.org.uk/
- The Gold Standards Framework Proactive Identification Guide: www.goldstandardsframework.org.uk/cd-content/uploads/files/PIG/NEW%20PIG%20-%20%20%2020.1.17%20KT%20vs17.pdf
- Preferred Priorities of Care (PPC): www.endoflifecare.nhs.uk

13   Safeguarding from Abuse and Neglect

■   WHAT IS ABUSE?

Abuse and neglect can encompass a range of acts, from apparently minor occurrences to criminal offences. Government guidance and local area policies on Safeguarding Adults identify seven different categories of abuse:

- physical abuse;
- sexual abuse;
- psychological or emotional abuse;
- neglect or acts of omission;
- financial or material abuse;
- discrimination;
- institutional abuse.

■   PEOPLE AT RISK OF ABUSE

- People with dementia are often classed as adults at risk of abuse (or 'vulnerable adults') under safeguarding processes and guidance, as they 'may be unable to protect themselves from significant harm or exploitation' (DoH 2000, updated 2015).
- People with dementia can experience many of the risk factors for abuse and neglect:
  - dependency on others for activities of daily living;
  - difficulties communicating with others;
  - cognitive impairment (difficulties with decision making);

DOI: 10.4324/9781003269946-13

- complex needs or behaviours that challenge others;
- social isolation;
- lack of specialist knowledge about their needs by those responsible for care.

■ WHY DOES ABUSE HAPPEN?

- Abuse can take place in any setting and can be carried out by anyone.
- It happens for many reasons, and often abusers do not identify that their actions might be considered abusive.
- Abuse or neglect can occur because a person does not know the correct approach, they are following out-of-date guidance or care plans or do not have the resources to carry out good care.
- Sometimes actions that are taken with the best of intentions (for example, to keep a person safe) can still result in an outcome that is abusive to the person with dementia.

■ BEING VIGILANT

- People with dementia will often not be able to report abuse or neglect in a straightforward manner because of their cognitive disabilities. Therefore it is vitally important that staff are vigilant to both verbal and non-verbal indicators of abuse and neglect.
- While the following could indicate something other than abuse or neglect, it should never be assumed that there is another explanation. Potential indicators, such as those below, should always be recorded and discussed in

accordance with your organisation's and local authority's safeguarding procedures:

- unexplained bruising and injury;
- poor nutritional status and dehydration;
- presence of restraints and locks;
- financial irregularities;
- negative interaction style, including telling off and rough handling;
- withdrawn, anxious, depressed, distressed or aggressive behaviours;
- lack of confidence or self-esteem.

■ TAKING ACTION

- All staff working with people with dementia have a responsibility to be aware of possible abuse and take appropriate action, wherever there is a concern that abuse may have taken place or may occur.
- All staff need to be aware of their professional codes of conduct and duty to respond appropriately to concerns of abuse and neglect
- All staff must know and follow their own organisation's and local authority's policies/procedures on safeguarding adults.

References

Abou-Saleh, M.T., Katona, C.L.E. and Kumar, A. (2011). *Principles and Practice of Geriatric Psychiatry*, 3rd edition. Chichester, John Wiley & Sons.

Age Concern (2006). *Hungry to be Heard: The scandal of malnourished older people in hospital*. London, Age Concern England.

Age Concern (2010). *Still Hungry to be Heard: The scandal of malnourished older people in hospital*. London, Age Concern England.

Alzheimer's Association (2021) Down Syndrome and Alzheimer's disease. Available at: www.alz.org/alzheimers-dementia/what-is-dementia/types-of-dementia/down-syndrome (accessed 27 October 2021)

Alzheimer's Disease International (2015). *World Alzheimer's Disease Report 2015: The global impact of dementia*. London, Alzheimer's Disease International.

Alzheimer's Society (UK) (2021). Demography information. Available at: http://alzheimers.org.uk/site/scripts/documents_info.php?documentID=412 (accessed 27 October 2021).

Blackhall, A., Hawkes, D., Hingley, D. and Wood, S. (2011). 'VERA framework: communicating with people who have dementia', *Nursing Standard* 26(10), 35–39.

Blossom, S. and Brayne, C. (2014). 'Prevalence and projections of dementia', in M. Downs, and B. Bowers (eds), *Excellence in Dementia Care: Research into practice*, 2nd edition (pp. 3–19). Maidenhead, Open University Press, McGraw Hill.

Brooker, D. and Latham, I. (2015). *Person-Centred Dementia Care Making Services Better*, 2nd edition. London, Jessica Kingsley.

Candy, B., Sampson, E.L. and Jones, L. (2009). 'Enteral feeding in older people with advanced dementia: findings from a Cochrane systematic review', *International Journal of Palliative Nursing* 15(8), 396–404.

Department of Health (2000, updated 2015). *No Secrets: Guidance on protecting vulnerable adults in care*. Available at www.gov.uk (accessed 27 October 2021).

Department of Health (2009). *Reference Guide to Consent for Examination or Treatment*, 2nd edition. London, Department of Health.

Gorelick, P.B. et al. (2011). 'Vascular contributions to cognitive impairment and dementia: a statement for healthcare professionals from the American Heart Association/American Stroke Association', *Stroke* 42, 2672–2713.

Jacoby, R., Dening, T. and Thomas, A. (2008). *Psychiatry in the Elderly*, 4th edition. Oxford, Oxford University Press.

Kitwood, T. (1997). *Dementia Reconsidered: The person comes first*. Maidenhead, Open University Press.

McKhann, G.M. et al. (2011). 'The diagnosis of dementia due to Alzheimer's disease: Recommendations from the National Institute on Aging and the Alzheimer's Association workgroup', *Alzheimer's & Dementia* 7(3), 263–269.

Mental Capacity Act (2005). Crown Copyright, Her Majesty's Stationery Office.

National Council for Palliative Care (NCPC) (2006). *Changing Gear: Guidelines for managing the last days of life in adults*. London, NCPC.

National Institute for Clinical Excellence (NICE) (2010). *Delirium, Clinical Guideline 103*. London, National Clinical Guidelines Centre.

National Institute for Clinical Excellence (NICE) (2018). *Clinical Guideline 97, Dementia assessment, management and support for people living with dementia and their families*. London, National Clinical Guidelines Centre.

National Institute for Clinical Excellence/Social Care Institute for Excellence (NICE–SCIE) (2006). *Clinical Guideline 42, Supporting people with dementia and their carers in Health and Social Care*. London, National Clinical Guidelines Centre.

National Institute for Health and Care Excellence (NICE) (2015). New guidelines to improve care for people at the end of life. Available at www.nice.org.uk (accessed 27 October 2021).

National Institute for Health and Clinical Excellence/Social Care Institute for Excellence (NICE–SCIE) (2007). *Clinical Guideline 42, Supporting people with dementia and their carers in Health and Social Care*. London, National Clinical Guidelines Centre.

Nuffield Council on Bioethics (2009). *Dementia: Ethical Issues*. London, Nuffield Council on Bioethics.

Office for National Statistics (2020). Leading causes of death. Available at www.ons.gov.uk (accessed 27 October 2021).

Royal College of Nursing (2019). *Commitment to the Care of People Living with Dementia SPACE Principles.* London, RCN.

SCIE (2021). *Person Centred Care.* Available at: www.scie.org.uk/prevention/choice/person-centred-care?gclid=EAlaIQobChMImYXr-7bq8wIVh49oCR2DVgaHEAAYASAAEglcQvD_BwE (accessed 27 October 2021)

Scofield, I. (2008). 'Delirium: challenges for clinical governance', *Journal of Nursing Management* 16, 127–133.

Sturdy, D., Heath, H., Ballard, C. and Burns, A. (2012). *Antipsychotic Drugs in Dementia: A best practice guide.* Harrow, Royal College of Nursing.

van der Steen, J.T. et al. on behalf of the European Association for Palliative Care (2014). White paper defining the optimal palliative care in older people with dementia: A Delphi study and recommendations from the European Association for Palliative Care. *Palliative Medicine* 28(3), 197–209.

Watson, R., MacDonald, J. and McReady, T. (2001). 'The Edinburgh Feeding Evaluation in Dementia Scale #2 (EdFED#2): inter- and intra-rater reliability', *Clinical Effectiveness in Nursing* 5(4), 184–186.

Wittenburg, R. et al. (2019). *Projections of Older People with Dementia and Cost of Dementia Care in the UK.* London, London School of Economics and Political Science.

Willoughby, J. (2012). 'Communicating with cognitively impaired patients', *Nursing Older People* 24(5), 14.